What Other Busy Moms Are Saying About GameChanger

"I worked out for MONTHS to get into shape for my wedding, 4-5 days per week. After just a month of working out just 3 days per week at GameChanger, I've seen amazing results rivaling those I saw for my wedding, with a lot less effort. Even my post-baby body was able to firm back up. The workouts at GameChanger are by far more efficient and effective than anything i've ever done!"

Lauren Novatkoski from Springfield, NJ

"I've been coming to GameChanger for close to two months now. I started out doing their Fit-Mom Program. As I got into it, I started to see results instantly and now I'm wearing jeans I never thought I'd fit into and literally just within two months of training at GameChanger."

Teri Kandel from Cranford, NJ

"The truth is after 30-days of working out at GameChanger's, I saw better results than working out with my personal trainer for a whole year. The coaches at GameChanger are always motivating and they make working out fun. I've never felt intimidated and I feel like they always bring me to the next level."

Kerri Solomine from Springfield, NJ

The Skinny Jeans Solution For Busy Moms

Chapter 1: The Skinny Jeans Solution For Busy Moms

Let's face the facts: getting back into your skinny jeans isn't an easy task. You're a busy mom who doesn't have time to spend hours in the gym. On top of that, you've been lied to from a lot of seemingly credible sources. These sources promise you the next best miracle pill or supplement, or a secret workout program that will transform your body instantly. Unfortunately, time after time, they fail to deliver.

Up until now, you might have thought it's your fault. The truth? Most companies are selling you products that flat-out don't work and are a big waste of money. After trying all the gadgets and gimmicks, you are left frustrated, while these big companies rake in huge profits.

Over the past 7 years, we've worked with hundreds of moms just like you who felt the same way. Luckily for them, they realized it's never too late to get the body they want. Like you, most of these women are busy moms who don't have a lot of time to workout. They were sick of all the hype being fed to them by companies who just wanted to make a quick

3   www.GameChangerGym.com

buck. They were tired of being led to believe it was their fault, because the crap they were buying wasn't working. They had enough of slaving away on cardio machines for hours each week, with little-to-no results to show for their hard work.

Throughout this book, our goal is to provide you with the right information you need to get the body you deserve. In the next few chapters, we'll share with you everything you need to know about getting back into those skinny jeans including: the best type of workouts to do on a tight schedule, super simple nutrition tweaks that will melt body fat, debunking the fat loss myths that are holding you back, and much more.

At the end, we'll offer four recommendations to help you make an informed decision when choosing a fitness program, and we'll give you five questions you should ask before joining.

Getting started at GameChanger is simple & easy. Go to gamechangergym.com/fitmom for more information on our Fit-Mom Program or email us directly at info@gamechangergym.com for more information.

Chapter 2: 5 Fat Loss Myths Exposed

There's a lot of confusing and frustrating information out there. With all of the "miracle" supplements, home DVDs, and fancy equipment, it's hard to know what's the *right* method for diet and exercise. Many of these companies and gurus are just trying to sell you something, and make bold claims to increase their popularity.

If you could transform your body so easily with these quick fixes, why haven't you gotten the results you want? Why is the rest of America so out of shape? This misinformation can leave you spinning your wheels, without the body you set out to achieve. Well, we're tired of your hard work and earned money going to waste. It's time to dispel these myths once and for all. Here are the 5 most common myths plaguing the fitness industry:

Myth #1: Cardio Burns More Fat Than Strength Training

One of the biggest misconceptions is that cardio is more effective for fat loss than strength training. Let's get something straight - the key to burning body fat is expending energy (aka burning calories), that part is true. Thus, it's understandable why you might think cardio is superior. However, strength training burns calories in ways you might not realize. Strength training is more effective for fat loss than cardio because when you strength train properly, you build lean muscle (muscle you cannot build by just doing cardio). The more lean muscle you have, the more calories you burn around the clock.

For example, if two people have the exact same daily activity, diet, genetics, and follow the same exercise program, the person with more lean muscle will burn more calories and thus have less body fat. Because she has less body fat and has more lean muscle, she will have a more toned and defined body.

You see, cardio builds hardly any lean muscle. So if you want to turn your body into a fat burning machine, you have to focus on proper strength training!

Strength training is also superior to cardio for calorie burning efficiency. As your body adapts to exercise, you'll burn fewer calories each time you do it. Thirty minutes of walking that used to burn 200 calories, will soon only burn 150 calories. With traditional slow cardio like this, the only variables you can change when your body adapts are the speed that you move and the time it takes you to run. As a busy parent, we know your time is precious, so increasing your treadmill walks or long distance runs from 30 minutes to 45, then to 60 and beyond is not an option.

Unlike cardio, with strength training there are so many variables. You can vary your sets, repetitions, weights, rest periods, equipment, and exercise variation when your body adapts, before ever having to increase your workout time. You can also incorporate sprints (10-30 seconds each), as they can generate muscle in your lower body similar to strength training. Because sprints are high intensity, you'll burn more calories in 20 minutes of sprints (including the rest between sprints) than you would with 30 minutes of non-stop, slow cardio work.

Since you can only exercise so much in a given week, getting the results you want is not just a function of how much fat or calories you burn when you're working out. The real secret is how metabolically active your body is the other 95%

of the time. Women with more lean muscle burn fat at a much greater rate than do those with less lean muscle- that's why these women are leaner, more toned, and defined.

Don't believe the myth that cardio burns more fat than strength training. Instead, understand that in order to tone up and define your body, you need to strength train!

Myth #2: Strength Training Makes You Big And Bulky

Have you ever heard that strength training will make you bulky? This is a big fat lie. In fact, just the opposite is true. Strength training will help you build lean muscle, giving you the tight and toned look you want. The more lean muscle you have, the more fat you burn. In other words, lean muscle is more compact and firmer than fat. So let's be clear about this - proper strength training will actually make you smaller, firmer, and more toned.

You see, women don't have the testosterone to add a lot of muscle mass. Men, on the other hand, gain mass and see exciting muscle growth through a surplus of calories and strength training. Let me explain this further -

testosterone is the principle male sex hormone, and it plays a major role in muscle growth. Most women naturally produce only a fraction of the testosterone that men have. This makes it impossible for a woman to increase her muscle size enough to look bulky or manly.

If you don't have enough muscle, no matter how much body fat you lose, chances are you will not see the changes in your body you were hoping for. That's because a toned body is one that has stripped off body fat to reveal and show off its lean muscle. The easiest way to build this lean muscle is through strength training. In the words of trainer and coach Nick Tumminello, "you can't build a perkier, rounder, or sexier *anything* without building muscle."

If you see a woman who appears too bulky, it's most likely because of excess body fat, *not* excess muscle mass. Strength training builds muscles, but excess calories cause fat gain, so it's safe to say improper nutrition is usually the culprit of a bulky physique.

Myth #3: You need to workout every day to lose fat

How many times have you stayed up late, searching for something on TV to put you to sleep, and you settle on a 30 minute infomercial of the latest exercise craze? Unfortunately, the fitness industry is filled with them. These programs usually entail a 60 minute long, non-stop workout, prescribed 7 days a week. The people doing the program get seemingly fantastic results. How can you pass on this program? It's time to pick up the phone, plunk down a one-time fee of a few hundred bucks, and finally get that cut six-pack and rock-hard glutes!

Then you realize you don't have time to workout 7 days a week, nor can you commit 60 minutes at a time away from your job or family. And the exercises seem like a lot of running and jumping around. You aren't made of glass, but you know some of those movements won't be friendly to your back or knees.

Even if you do commit to this program, these intense workouts are too taxing and time consuming to stick with long-term. You'll have spent all that time, money, and effort, and in a few months you'll be right back where you started.

You were promised a better body and fast results, but it's been taken away so quickly. You can't dedicate all that time and energy into these workouts. How are you supposed to shed those unwanted pounds?

The Key to Permanently Losing Body Fat

Fortunately, the message that you must perform intense exercise for 400+ minutes a week is a myth. The solution for losing weight is simple: it's the age-old formula of calories-in vs. calories-out. If you burn more calories than you take in, you'll lose weight. If you take in more calories than you burn, you'll gain weight. That's the magic   solution!

"How do I use this formula?" is what you're probably asking yourself. You burn more calories through exercise, and you take in fewer by eating higher quality food. You do *not* need to workout every day to get the body you want. In fact, most of the moms that train with us at GameChanger workout only 3-4 days a week for 45 minutes, and their results speak for themselves. The key to their success is proper strength training. You can't go to the gym and just use a few machines or very light dumbbells that don't challenge you.

Remember, the more lean muscle you have, the more calories you'll burn throughout the whole day - even when you're sleeping, working, and while taking care of your family! The best part is, the more lean muscle you have, the less you have to exercise to burn those calories. And the way you achieve this is with 3-4 proper strength training sessions a week.

So get off the hamster wheel and stop doing endless hours of cardio a week. You're a busy mom with a family to take care of. You don't have hours to waste in the gym. Why workout more than necessary to get results? More isn't always better. Instead, focus on the quality of your workouts rather than the quantity.

Myth #4: Women should only lift for high reps to lose fat

The same people who say strength training will make you big and bulky will also tell you to do high rep training to sculpt and tone your muscles. The truth is, the only way to "tone" and "sculpt" your muscles is through *building* new lean muscle! The idea that you can shape your muscles with high rep training is a big fat lie.

The problem with high rep training and why it won't help you get the results you want is the weight you're lifting isn't challenging enough. Think about it this way: if you use 5lb dumbbells for an exercise, is that any different from lifting your pocket book? We've yet to hear any women brag about how fit they got from carrying around their purses! Did you lose body fat from carrying your 10lb children around when they were still babies? The answer is probably no.

You'll get a toned body from shedding body fat, and having firm, lean muscle to show off. If your only exercise is training with light weights and very high reps, you won't provide enough stimulation to produce any tone in your physique.

Extremely light weight training is no different from everyday tasks you're already doing like playing with your kids, carrying groceries, or moving things around the house. It you haven't gotten results by moving light weights around throughout the whole day, why do more of it? Maybe it's time for a change.

Exercise That Works

The key to a proper strength training program is using compound exercises that work multiple muscle groups simultaneously. This is best for giving you a toned look, as well as burning the most calories in the least amount of time. Lifting very light weights for many repetitions could even burn *fewer* calories than heavier training since each rep doesn't require much energy. Light weights won't get you toned, and they can be inefficient!

This does not mean you have to lift the heaviest weight you possibly can. The weight should be heavy enough to challenge you, but moderate enough that you'll have energy for an entire 45 minute workout. This usually keeps you with repetitions between 6 and 15 for each exercise. If you can't achieve 6 reps, try going lighter. If you can get 15 reps with an exercise, it's time to use a heavier weight.

There's no perfect weight or number of reps for fat loss, but one thing is certain: you need to challenge your body and get out of your comfort zone to burn fat and earn your way into skinny jeans!

Myth #5: You can just eat less to lose fat

There are tons of popular diet protocols that work: Atkins; South Beach; Zone; Paleo; Isagenix; Nutrisystem; Medifast; Jenny Craig, to just name a few. These diets take different approaches, but they all have one thing in common: they force you to eat fewer calories.

That's why they work! They don't use magical shakes, foods, or nutrients. They don't cleanse you of harmful toxins (only your liver and kidney can do that). They don't improve your hormones.

So armed with this information, all you have to do to lose fat is eat *less*, right? This appears true on the surface, but there's a problem with this approach: a restrictive diet is not sustainable.

The popular diets I mentioned have produced many successful transformations, but how many people also tried these diets and *didn't* get the results they wanted? How many people couldn't stick to the diet because of unrealistic guidelines, periods of starvation, or expensive shakes they had to drink? Also, did the people who experienced these transformations sustain these changes long after they finished the diet?

www.GameChangerGym.com

Anytime you go on a diet, you'll eventually go off of it, and chances are you'll gain all the weight back and then some. We've all been on the never-ending roller coaster ride that happens with fad and restrictive diets.

The key is to never go on a diet in the first place. Instead, you need to find a balanced lifestyle that allows you to eat the foods you enjoy, while getting the results you want. Don't start a diet: begin a new lifestyle that includes strength training and a healthy way of eating that you can envision yourself doing for the rest of your life.

Also, if you reduce calories too drastically with a fad type diet, you'll create new problems:

3 Reasons Why Fad Diets Don't Work

Fad diets can bring rapid weight loss. Unfortunately, this rapid weight loss comes at a cost.

Binging: Eating a very low calorie diet can cause hunger to skyrocket, leading to overeating. These binges can compromise your fat loss and discourage you from sticking with your fat loss program. Binging isn't a matter of lack-of will power. If you put your body under too much stress, you will lose control sooner or later, regardless of how strong-willed you think you are.

Burn _Fewer_ Calories: Your body fights you every step of the way as you diet, doing its best to maintain its body weight (no wonder fat loss is so hard!). This was useful for most of human history when food and shelter were scarce and extra body fat helped us survive. It's less welcomed when trying to fit into an old dress, a new bathing suit, or skinny jeans. As you eat less, your body burns fewer calories. Cut calories too low and you'll burn too few calories to make fat loss manageable. There needs to be a fine balance of eating less, while giving your body enough fuel to burn calories.

Lose Weight But Keep The Flab: Eating less does not solve the challenge of developing muscle tone and giving you something to show-off. Exercise is just as important to transforming your body as nutrition. If you neglect strength training and simply eat less, your body weight might decrease, but your belly fat will not. If you don't lose the flab, chances are you won't be happy with what you see in the mirror.

Chapter 3: The # 1 Ingredient For Fat Loss

The most impactful ingredient for fat loss isn't a special diet pill or "superfood" you need to buy at the local farmers market. It's not something you need to take, but rather something to eliminate...liquid calories!

Eliminating liquid calories from your diet is one of the fastest ways to shed pounds. Drinking these fluids is an easy way to amass hundreds of calories without becoming full. Over the past 10 years, a number of studies have found associations between sugar sweetened beverages and long-term weight gain.

Which calorie-dense beverages are expanding your waistline?

Avoid These 7 Fat Inducing Drinks
1. Soda (non-diet)
2. Juice
3. Gatorade
4. Energy drinks
5. Vitamin Water
6. Coffee from popular chains
7. Alcohol

1. Soda (non-diet)

This is no secret. If you drink soda, eliminating it from your diet is the first change you should make! The average 12 oz can of soda has about 140 calories and 38 grams of sugar. If you're ordering from a fast food place or restaurant, you're likely to drink a much larger portion.

2. Juice

The next candidate on our list is not so obvious. Isn't juice simply fruit in liquid form? Isn't juice healthy, especially if it's 100% fruit juice? We've heard brands like Ocean Spray and Tropicana extol the virtues of their juice for years. Those beverages have got to be a healthy choice!

Here's a closer look at popular fruit juice brands, per 12 fluid ounces. Remember, the average can of soda has 140 calories and 38g of sugar.

Product	Calories	Sugar
Ocean Spray Classic Cranberry Juice	163 calories	39g sugar
Tropicana 100% Orange Juice	165 calories	40g sugar
Naked Mango	225 calories	54g sugar

Welch's 100% Grape Juice	210 calories	54g sugar
Mott's Original 100% Apple Juice	180 calories	43g sugar
Minute Maid Fruit Punch	135 calories	37g sugar

Every single juice listed has more calories and sugar per fluid ounce than soda! All except for Minute Maid Fruit Punch, which saves you an entire 5 calories and 1 gram of sugar- that's equivalent to one piece of sugar free gum.

The most damning nutrition fact of most fruit juices is they contain zero grams of fiber. Most whole fruits have adequate fiber, and when fiber is lost as they're processed into juice, they lose part of their health benefits. We'll learn more later about the importance of fiber in your diet.

3. Gatorade

Gatorade is very popular among athletes, and focuses its marketing campaign on its high electrolyte content to keep you hydrated. Before you feel the need to bring a bottle of Gatorade to every workout session, let's learn a few more facts:

A) The average bottle is 20 oz and contains 130 calories and 34g of sugar, similar to our soda can.

B) Unless you live in the sweltering heat with no air conditioning, play competitive sports for hours at a time, or have a pre-existing medical condition, regular water will keep you plenty hydrated!

Water gives most people the same benefits as Gatorade but without the calories. In fact, the 2006 film *Idiocracy* did a fantastic job satirizing the over-hyped benefits of electrolyte drinks for everyday people. The movie takes place 500 years into the future in a dystopian society where advertising dominates, and the American people are grossly unintelligent. The fictional sports drink Brawndo is the drink of choice and is even used to water crops, because it has electrolytes and "it's got what plants crave!" Brawndo could not grow the crops, but Gatorade can grow your waistline.

4. Energy Drinks

People are busier than ever, so it's no shock that energy drinks (most are stronger and sweeter than a cup of coffee) are flying off the shelves. Brands like Red Bull and Monster have taken off, keeping people of all ages stimulated and awake for sports, work, school, and other activities that require your undivided attention. This caffeinated goodness comes at a price- similar calorie and sugar contents to soda, juice, and sports drinks.

5. Vitamin Water

Most people lack the recommended servings of many vitamins and minerals in their diets, so they supplement with a multi-vitamin pill. Vitamin Water delivers these vitamins in a more palatable way. Once again, the tasty beverage is not much different from soda in its sugar content. Stick to whole food sources for your vitamin and mineral needs. Supplement with a multi-vitamin pill if you're worried your food isn't doing the job.

6. Coffee

Coffee itself has many benefits, but it doesn't take much to turn it into a calorie dense beverage that is making you fat. Sugar additives can make your morning cup of Joe higher in calories than a typical soda, particularly if you're getting it from a popular coffee franchise. Here are a few examples:

Dunkin' Donuts Coffee- Calorie Content per 14 oz (Medium) from dunkindonuts.com

Caramel Latte w/ milk	350 Calories
Caramel Mocha Latte w/ milk	330 Calories
Most Flavored Lattes w/ skim milk	270 Calories

Starbucks Coffee: Calorie Content per 12 oz (Tall) from Starbucks.com

Double Chocolaty Chip Creme Frappuccino	200 Calories
Iced Espresso Classics Cafe Mocha	140 Calories
Double Shot Energy Coffee Drink	210 Calories
Caffe Latte Espresso	190 Calories
Caffe Mocha Espresso	290 Calories
Caramel Flan Latte Espresso	250 Calories
Caramel Macchiato Espresso	240 Calories
Cinnamon Dolce Latte Espresso	260 Calories

Flavored Latte Espresso-	250 Calories
Cinnamon Dolce Frappuccino	260 Calories

This information is even more eye-opening when you consider that many people order larger sizes than a 12 oz Tall from Starbucks or a 14 oz medium from Dunkin' Donuts, and this doesn't include the milk and sugar you add. A medium (Grande) Caffe Latte Espresso from Starbucks would actually be 250 calories, rather than the 190 listed for the small size.

How many people do you know that might be having more than one of these beverages a day? If you drink two of these espressos from Starbucks, that's 500 extra calories you don't even notice! An additional 500 calories in your diet a day can have you gain 1lb a week.

7. Alcohol

Like it or not, alcoholic drinks have calories. You don't need to swear them off to fit into those skinny jeans, but you need to monitor your intake. Here's a look at calorie information of popular alcohol drink brands:

1.5 oz Jose Cuervo Tequila	98 calories
1.5 oz Seagrams Gin	104 calories
5 oz Red Wine	125 calories
12 oz Bud Light	110 calories
12 oz Blue Moon	170 calories
11.2 oz Mike's Hard Lemonade-	220 calories

A closer look shows wine and beer are not so different from a can of Coke. Think about what this means if you drink wine a few times per week, or every night, or multiple glasses a night.

You have even more to contend with in mixed drinks:

- A shot of whiskey is 98 calories, and what if you're having Jack and Coke? Now you're drinking additional calories from soda.
- If you choose a Gin and Tonic, don't forget the 120 calories in each can of Seagrams Tonic Water.
- If you're having margaritas, you need to account for the calories from the tequila

as well as the 120 calories in 4 ounces of your margarita mix.

This means most mixed drinks are equivalent to 1-2 cans of soda!

Alcohol further complicates your skinny jeans solution because when you drink it, it's usually with extra food. A study performed in 2001 suggests alcohol stimulates hunger, and another study from this year (2015) concludes "moderate alcohol consumption increased subsequent food intake, specifically of high-fat savory foods".

You have a lot going on in your life. You deserve to relax, unwind, and have fun. Understand that if you plan on drinking alcohol while trying to lose or maintain your body weight, the process is a little more challenging. We recommend you limit yourself to 2-3 drinks per week.

Replacing Liquid Calories

Eliminating these drinks doesn't mean you have to drink *less.* Our first recommendation is something you already know: drink more water! Drinking more water can be the missing component of your nutrition to speed along your fat loss.

Why Water Works

Drinking water, particularly before a big meal, helps you feel fuller. The more water you drink, the more likely you are to eat fewer calories.

A study in 2010 tested this principle. It compared two groups of dieters who were given a meal plan of equal calories. The only difference: one group drank 500ml of water before each meal. At the end of 12 weeks, the group that drank water before each meal "showed a 44% greater decline in weight" than the non-water group!

Another study from May 2015 even indicates the amount of water women intake is positively associated with their mood!

A great goal to aim for is to drink half of your body weight in ounces of water each day. If you weigh 150lbs, that's 75 oz of water, or almost 4.5 standard bottles of Poland Spring. If that is a drastic increase from your current intake, drink more than you do now, and slowly work up to the half-your-body-weight goal. Don't underestimate the impact that something as simple as water can have on your health and body.

Most of what you drink should be water, but you don't have to rely on it exclusively. You can also use non-calorie liquids.

Skinny Jeans Approved Drink List

- ➤ Coffee w/ approved additives
- ➤ Tea
- ➤ Seltzer
- ➤ Artificially Sweetened Beverages:
  - Diet Soda
  - Diet Snapple
  - Vitamin Water Zero
  - G2 series Gatorade
  - Crystal Light

1. Coffee

We know what you're thinking- isn't coffee one of the fat inducing drinks? It turns into one at popular coffee chains, but coffee itself is skinny jeans approved. Long-term coffee consumption is associated with a decreased risk of Type II Diabetes, along with other health benefits. Many people believe the caffeine in coffee helps suppress appetite. Caffeine also *slightly* boosts metabolism.

Limit yourself to 1-2 tbsp of creamer/milk and 1-2 tsp of sugar/sweetener per cup. Put in these additives yourself, or make sure to give your server clear instructions.

2. Tea

Tea is in the same boat as coffee. It can be a harmless, soothing beverage, or you can turn it into a gut-growing milkshake. Follow the same milk and sugar guidelines as coffee. Tea is a great choice to have between meals or late at night before bed.

3. Seltzer

It's simply carbonated water. Sometimes it has a little sodium, sometimes not. Either way, it's a perfectly acceptable beverage, and can satisfy your taste buds like soda.

4. Artificially Sweetened Beverages

We know what you've heard- they cause cancer, diabetes, brain damage, and even weight *gain*. They're unnatural, unsafe, and illegal in some countries. Diet soda, Splenda, and aspartame should be avoided at all costs.

Here's the unabashed truth: You've been lied to. Zero calorie sweeteners like aspartame are completely safe for humans. Irresponsible journalists and misinformed doctors have spread false information. They use fear mongering to draw attention to themselves, with no regard for the real scientific facts.

There's no need to worry about having artificial sweeteners in moderation. Scientists have studied them for years, and the vast majority of evidence shows they are safe. There have been over 100 studies proving aspartames' safety in particular.

Not only is the evidence too much to ignore, but almost EVERY important medical and health organization claims legal artificial sweeteners, namely aspartame, are safe. The following government and non-profit organizations all approve aspartame use for humans: FDA; National Cancer Institute; World Health Organization; European Union; Health Canada; Food Standards Australia New Zealand; American Cancer Society; American Diabetes Association; American Heart Association; Mayo Clinic; Academy of Nutrition Dietetics; American Academy of Family Physicians; American Council on Science and Health; Alzheimer's Association; Asthma and Allergy Foundation of America; National Multiple Sclerosis Society.

That's a lot of support to ignore! Media outlets irresponsibly report poorly constructed studies claiming artificially sweetened beverages are dangerous- probably to peak interest and boost ratings. Listen to the crowd that knows what it's talking about, like the scientific and medical community. If drinking zero calorie-sweetened beverages helps you replace calorie-filled liquids, go for it!

Use these beverages to make your meals more filling, stop hunger between meals, or replace dessert. Like all things, enjoy them in moderation.

Getting started at GameChanger is simple & easy.

Go to gamechangergym.com/fitmom for more information on our Fit-Mom Program or email us directly at info@gamechangergym.com for more information.

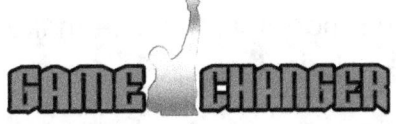

Chapter 4: Slowly Add This One Thing To Your Meal to Burn Fat Around The Clock

Did you know you don't always need to eat less to lose weight? That's because not all calories are created equal.

In fact, you can actually add something to your diet to help you burn more fat. Increasing your protein intake will help you burn off calories while your body digests it. This is known as the thermic effect of food.

Our bodies don't only burn calories when we move - our bodies burn calories during processes that occur even when we rest. One of those processes is digestion. When we digest protein, we burn even MORE calories!

More protein also helps you burn calories throughout the day because it builds lean muscle mass. Remember what we learned earlier? Having more lean muscle makes your body burn more calories!

Eat More Protein, Avoid More Snacking

Protein helps control your appetite. Protein is more satiating than carbohydrates or fat, so if your meal has more protein, you'll stay fuller for longer. If you get hungry soon after a meal, you probably didn't eat enough protein.

Part of the reason people snack throughout the day is their meals are comprised mainly of carbs and fat. Most Americans only have a high protein meal at dinner. If people would eat more protein for breakfast and lunch, they might not be so hungry during the day.

Neglecting protein in the morning can set you up for a day of poor nutrition. Your low-protein breakfast doesn't keep you full, so you take an early lunch. Your early lunch leaves you hungry hours before dinner time, so you visit the vending machine or have a snack with your afternoon coffee. Or the coffee has so much sugar in it that it's a snack itself. Whatever the case, lack of protein led to hunger, which made you eat too many calories.

Studies continuously show high protein diets produce more weight loss than standard protein diets. They might even improve blood pressure and blood sugar levels, though more research needs to be done.

Use this information to your advantage by increasing your daily protein intake. You'll burn more calories and stay fuller longer!

Skinny Jeans Recommended Protein Sources

- Lean chicken breast
- 90% or leaner beef
- Turkey
- Fish, oysters, and other seafood
- Ham
- Low-fat or fat-free dairy
- Eggs, egg whites, and egg beaters
- Tofu
- Soy beans and protein powder
- Whey protein powder
- Protein bars

It's important to distinguish these foods from other meat sources like: burgers; sausage; meatballs; hot dogs; chicken wings and fried chicken; bacon; pepperoni; salami; bologna, to name a few. Those animal sources often have more fat than protein per serving.

Meat Source	Fat (g)	Protein (g)
Kirkland Beef Hot Dog	14	8
Ballpark Burger	19	14
Premio Sausage	14	12
Tyson Bacon, 2 slices	7	5
Pepperoni	11	6
Hormel Genoa Salami	18	11
Boar's Head Bologna	13	7

If you're craving these foods, look for leaner versions like turkey bacon, turkey pepperoni, and 90% or leaner burgers or hot dogs. Look for the protein content to be about double (or more) of the fat content.

Even protein bars can be deceiving- many of them are glorified candy bars. If a protein bar doesn't have around 10% of its calories in grams of protein, then it's *not* a real protein bar. That means if it has 200 calories, it should have about 20g of protein.

Bar	Protein(g)	Calories
Quest Chocolate Chip Cookie Dough	21	190
MetRx Big 100 Colossal	31	410
FiberOne Protein Caramel Nut	7	130
Kind PB Dark Chocolate Protein Plus	7	200
Pure Protein Chocolate Deluxe	21	180
Supreme Protein Caramel Nut Choc	30	360
Special K Strawberry Protein	10	170

- The Kind Protein Plus bar, FiberOne bar, and Special K protein bar are low in protein. These brands added more protein into these bars than in their standard bars, but they still aren't significant sources of protein.

- MetRx and Supreme Protein bars have 30 grams of protein, but at more than 300 calories each they don't hit the 10% rule. That means that rest of the calories are coming from significant carbs and fat.

This isn't bad for a meal, but it's not what we recommend for protein supplementation.

- Quest Nutrition and Pure Protein exceed our 10% rule, since they both have 20g of protein for less than 200 calories. These are good bets for protein bars.

Foods Masquerading as High Protein Sources

- Nuts
- Nut butters like peanut butter, almond butter
- Regular yogurt
- Whole Milk
- Beans
- Quinoa

These foods are *not* very high in protein. They are fine food sources and can be part of a healthy and balanced diet. They provide some protein and give you good protein *in addition* to the sources mentioned before, but they aren't *high* protein sources for your meals.

Food	Protein(g)	Calories
Planters Peanuts, 1 oz	7	170
Almonds, 1 oz	6	165
Skippy Peanut Butter, 1 tbsp	3.5	95
Activia Yogurt, 4oz	4	110
Whole Milk	8	140
Black Beans, ½ cup	7	110
Kidney Beans	6	95
Chickpeas, canned 4 oz	5.5	135
Quinoa, 1 oz	4	110

Include these foods in your diet if you enjoy them. They have healthy fats, some are high in fiber, and the dairy products are high in essential minerals. But don't rely on them to be your main protein source at a meal.

How Much Protein Should I Have a Day?

Aim for 1 gram of protein per pound of your goal body weight. So if you currently weigh 175lbs and want to lose 25lbs, putting you at 150lbs, aim for 150g of protein a day. Think of a palm-sized portion (or 4oz) of a protein source as 25 grams of protein. This means six servings of protein a day for your goals.

Our guideline probably means eating more protein than you're used to. Slowly build up to it. If your goal weight means eating six servings of protein a day but you currently eat three, only increase to four. After a week or two of sticking to this habit, increase to five. Once you've mastered that, you're ready for six.

Another strategy for tracking your protein intake is to keep a food log or track your daily intake using an app like My Fitness Pal. Track your food for three days and figure out your current daily protein intake. Then track for another 3 days and try to reach the gram-per-body-weight goal.

Easy Ways To Increase Your Protein Intake by Meal

Breakfast: Eggs or egg whites, any style, are the ticket to a high protein, nutritious breakfast. If you're too busy to sit down for breakfast, blend up a delicious smoothie with whey protein powder, fruit, and unsweetened almond milk.

Lunch: Ditch the sandwich or wrap for a big salad. Make up for the missing bread by doubling the meat in your salad.

Dinner: Replace half your processed carbs at dinner with a protein source. For example, if you're having chicken and rice, replace half of your normal rice portion with chicken. There won't be less food on your plate, but you'll get more protein!

Snacks/Dessert: Swap out ice cream for a frozen Greek yogurt bar.

Any Time- Use protein powder as a replacement for any meal or snack. Most powders give you 25g of protein for just 1 scoop, 120 calories of almost exclusively protein! It's very convenient for busy people. It doesn't require cooking, prep time, nor a table to sit down at. Put a scoop in a shaker bottle, add water, shake it up, and you're ready to drink it. Protein powders come in a variety of sweet flavors. If you have a few minutes, make a protein smoothie by blending up protein powder, fruit, ice, and almond milk or water. You can even add protein powder to your oatmeal, cereal, or coffee in the morning. The possibilities for protein powder are almost endless!

Getting started at GameChanger is simple & easy.

Go to gamechangergym.com/fitmom for more information on our Fit-Mom Program or email us directly at info@gamechangergym.com for more information.

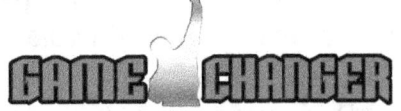

Chapter 5: Fill Up On This For Faster Fat Loss

No matter how "good" your diet is, it won't work if you're constantly hungry. If you control your cravings and stay full, you have a much better chance of getting the body you want! Add more fiber into your diet to keep that full feeling in your stomach long after meals.

Avoid an Empty Stomach, Cravings, & Grogginess Throughout Your Day

Fiber is a non-digestible carbohydrate. Fibrous carbs don't have as many calories as other carbohydrates. This is why nutritionists recommend complex carbohydrates over simple carbohydrate sources - because they contain more fiber.

High Fiber Sources for Skinny Jeans
- Vegetables: particularly dark green sources
- Beans: black, kidney, green peas, Lima, garbanzo (chick peas), lentils, pinto
- Nuts and nut butters (not nut oils, like peanut oil)
- Avocado

- Fruit: particularly berries, apples, bananas, oranges
- Potatoes: particularly sweet potatoes
- Whole grains: bran and high-fiber cereal brands, some whole grain breads and wraps, oats, whole wheat pasta

Many of these high fiber sources are the same foods mistakenly identified as high in protein. This should make something clear: most foods can have a place in your diet, it just depends on the context. For example, adding avocado to your meal will give you more fiber, but not a whole lot more protein. So if you need more fiber for the day, it's an excellent choice. If you've had plenty of fiber but need more protein and fewer calories, skip the avocado this time and add a lean protein source.

Don't Avoid Greens If You Want Skinny Jeans!

Make vegetables a priority at every lunch and dinner. Since so many of the carbs in vegetables are from fiber, they have very few calories *and* keep you fuller longer- talk about a winning combination. Your parents told you your whole life vegetables keep you healthy- maybe they forgot to preach their fat slashing effects!

Take a look at how many ounces of vegetables it takes to reach 100 calories. Keep in mind, 16 ounces is one pound:

Vegetable	Ounces Per 100 Calories (raw)
Kale	7
Onion	8.4
Carrot	8.6
Broccoli	10.4
Green Beans	11.4
Cauliflower	14.1
Eggplant	14.7
Spinach	15.3
Mushroom	16
Asparagus	17.6
Green Pepper	17.7
Tomato	19.5
Romaine Lettuce	20.7
Squash/Zucchini	22
Cucumber	22

Compare that to the portion sizes of other carb sources to reach 100 calories:

Carbohydrate	Ounces Per 100 Calories
Oreo cookie	0.75
Doughnut (plain)	0.8
Quaker Oatmeal (dry)	0.9
Cheerios cereal	1
Pasta (dry)	1
Muffin (plain)	1.2
Bread (white or wheat)	1.4
Breyer's Ice Cream	1.6
White Rice	2.7
Brown Rice	3.7
White Potato	3.7
Sweet Potato (baked)	3.9

17.6 oz asparagus and 1 oz pasta have the same calories, but which will keep you fuller and prevent you from snacking? We'll take our chances with the pound of asparagus!

If you aren't as hungry, you'll have less trouble sticking to your nutrition plan. No one expects you to eat a pound of vegetables for dinner, but the point is this: Replace some of your carbs with vegetables and you'll feel fuller while eating fewer calories.

If you don't like asparagus, choose a vegetable you do like. If you think you don't like vegetables, keep trying new ones. There are so many to choose from! Try combining a few different ones, use calorie free condiments like soy sauce, or add different herbs and spices. Grill, bake, or boil them. Buy them fresh or frozen. Another strategy is to have at least one large salad a day. Use either 2 servings of a low-fat dressing, or oil and vinegar with no more than 1 tbsp of olive oil.

The lesson: don't worry about which vegetables you choose or how you prepare them. As long as you aren't lathering them with oil or barbecue sauce, you'll get the benefits.

Fiber Recommendations

Aim to have a *minimum* of 1% of your total daily calories in grams of fiber. Put simply: if you eat 1,500 calories a day, have at least 15g of fiber a day. That's a minimum recommendation, try to have even more.

When you go grocery shopping, make sure most of your carb sources have at least 10% of their carbs from fiber. That means if you're purchasing whole wheat bread and it has 20g of carbs per slice, it better have at least 2g of fiber. Look at food labels, educate yourself, and you'll have better success.

Since you've read this far, we'll let you in on a little secret: fiber can counterbalance the negative effects of sugar. As long as you hit your daily fiber goal and don't consume too many calories, you can fit a sugary treat into your diet without negative repercussions to your health and physique!

Additional Skinny Jeans Solutions To Prevent Cravings

1. Eat Slowly

When you begin eating, it takes time to feel full. You won't feel satisfied until you get further away from that first bite. If you eat slowly, you'll have eaten less food in that time frame. Try taking 15-20 minutes to finish a meal, but if that seems too long, simply eat your food slower than you currently do. Sit down during your meals, focus on what you're eating, and take time to enjoy it. Another skinny jeans tip: the warmer your food is, the slower you'll eat.

2. Fill Half of Your Plate with Veggies

Vegetables provide very few calories for a lot of food. Fill *at least* half of your plate with vegetables. If you commit to polishing them off before your other food, you might not want that second helping of pasta, or even dessert.

3. Choose Berries and Melons

Fruits have many of the same health benefits as vegetables, but they provide a lot more calories. If you want the best bang-for-your-buck to get the nutrients and taste of fruit but for fewer calories, try berries and melon. Strawberries, blueberries, and cranberries have more fiber than most fruit, and also have fewer calories per serving than fruits like apples, bananas, and oranges. For instance, 6 ounces of blueberries is a bigger portion than a medium sized banana, yet they have roughly the same calories. An ounce of melon (watermelon, cantaloupe, honeydew) contains fewer calories than an ounce of most other fruits.

Stop Avoiding Fruit

Some people are afraid to eat fruit when they're trying to slim down. I've even heard one popular nutrition guru refer to fruit as "watery candy" and "bags of sugar." When you hear someone say mindless statements like this, it's time to run, hide, and never look back.

Fruit should be part of any healthy, balanced diet. Along with vegetables, it has vitamins and minerals that prevent illness, and there's research to back this up.

The sugar in fruit concerns dieters, specifically the fructose. You've probably heard people label high fructose corn syrup (HFCS) as a main contributor to obesity. The average recommended limit of fructose for adults is about 50 grams a day. To put this into context, a medium sized banana has 7g of fructose, and two cups of strawberries have 4g. That means you'd have to eat 4 bananas and 16 cups of strawberries A DAY to reach the 50g limit. That's a lot of fruit!

You'll gain weight from eating fruit the same way you'll gain weight from eating *any* food - by eating too many calories. Is it easy to overeat enough fruit to gain weight? Not according to the research. A study from the American Society of Nutrition published in 2015 suggests a higher fruit intake for women is associated with a *lower* risk of weight gain.

Don't Fill Up on This

It's smart to eat foods packed with essential nutrients, but the key is always moderation. Remember, too many calories of ANYTHING leads to too much body fat. What foods are healthy but easy to overeat? Here are some of the usual suspects:

1. Olive Oil

You've probably heard people refer to olive oil as a "good fat", and this is true as it's a good source of monounsaturated fats. But too much of a good thing can be a problem. Just one tablespoon of olive oil has 14g of fat and 120 calories. If you're using olive oil and vinegar as your salad dressing and not measuring out your portion, think about how easy it is for your salad to transform from "healthy" into "unhealthy".

2. Coconut Oil

It's become very trendy to add coconut oil to drinks like smoothies, protein shakes, and coffee. Coconut oil has the same calorie profile as olive oil - 120 per table spoon. If you're adding coconut oil to a beverage, measure it out, and cap it at one per day.

3. Nuts

Nuts are a great snack option. They are a source of both healthy fats and fiber, and are a great flavor-enhancer for your meals. However, they have the same calorie-dense problem as olive oil. Just one ounce of nuts has nearly 170 calories and 15g of fat. If you're snacking on nuts without monitoring your portion size, it's easy to eat more than a few ounces without realizing it. Keep nuts as part of your diet, but stick to moderate portion sizes.

Go to gamechangergym.com/fitmom for more information on our Fit-Mom Program or email us directly at info@gamechangergym.com for more information.

Chapter 6: Burn More Fat In Only 45 Minutes With This Simple Type Of Workout

You've had trouble changing your body, but you're not alone. The good news is - it's not your fault. Up until now, you've been given the wrong tools to be successful and sculpt your body. You have the desire and dedication, you just need the proper workout method to get the results you want.

We've discussed the need for strength training to get the body you deserve. Once you've become familiar with the movements of strength training and developed a solid base for your body, it's time to take your physique to the next level with strength training that's even more geared toward your goals as a fit mom. This type of workout is called *metabolic* strength training!

Metabolic strength training uses traditional strength training with a few modifications to make fat loss the ultimate goal. Contrary to popular belief, you don't need to workout for hours on end to get the body you want, and you don't have to suffer through slow, boring cardio workouts. You can get all the exercise you need in 45 minutes, only a few times a week, using this style of training.

Metabolic strength training incorporates challenging weight lifting, body weight training, and cardiovascular work to burn fat, while toning your body! This training uses full body exercises and challenging weights to give you the most "bang for your buck." This means you will burn more calories in less time. And if you're a busy mom, one of your most valuable and limited assets is your time!

The Missing Component To Toning, Sculpting, And Defining Your Muscles

With metabolic strength training, you can perform 5-7 total exercises to target your entire physique in only 45 minutes. You'll use dumbbells, barbells, and your own body weight. Take enough rest (1-2 minutes) between movements to keep up your strength, but not enough to bring your heart rate down to its normal resting rate. Doing this type of workout along with sound nutrition will give you better, longer-lasting, and safer results than a typical fat loss program.

Typical fat loss style workouts usually fall into one of two categories:

1. Chaotic, Fast Paced Workouts (often seen in infomercials)

2. Long-Distance Running

1. The fast-paced workouts are usually chaotic and highly impact your joints. High intensity workouts are great for fat loss, but performing movements without enough recovery or proper form can wreak havoc on your body. Even body weight movements like squats, lunges, push-ups, and especially jumps can be dangerous if you're too fatigued or use poor technique.

2. Long distance running burns calories, but doesn't give your body any definition. If the only exercise you do is long distance cardio, you'll position your physique to become the dreaded "skinny-fat." And because your body is moving so slowly with long distance running, you need to do LOTS of it to burn enough calories. Also, slow cardio only burns calories *while* you do it. Strength training builds lean muscle mass that burns more calories throughout the whole day!

What you'll love most about metabolic strength training is the variety! You can change up your exercises as often as you want by varying the tempo, equipment, and repetitions. You can switch between barbells, dumbbells, resistance bands, or your own body weight. Perform movements while standing, sitting, or in different positions on the ground. Vary the speed of your repetitions. The exercise possibilities are endless!

It's imperative to enjoy your workouts. The best workout routine isn't one that makes you sweat most, makes you tired, or is necessarily the most popular. The best workout style is the one you will stick to.

Think about the exercise you've done before: lots of walking and running, home workout videos, yoga, pilates, etc. These forms of exercise have their place, but did they get you the body you want? How often did you have to do them? Did you enjoy them and continue doing them for long periods of time? Did it keep you injury free? Your style of exercise needs to meet all of these criteria for it to improve your health and fitness.

Good nutrition and cardio exercise are not enough to give you the tone and definition you deserve. Metabolic strength training will tone your body in a way you've never experienced before! You won't truly appreciate the benefits until you actually begin training. Your clothes will fit better. You'll appreciate parts of your body that you never even thought about before. Strength training will sculpt your body to set you apart from women who shy away from weight training. This is your chance to not only make progress, but also to have the courage to do what most people won't, and you'll be rewarded for it.

Getting started at GameChanger is simple & easy.

Go to gamechangergym.com/fitmom for more information on our Fit-Mom Program or email us directly at info@gamechangergym.com for more information.

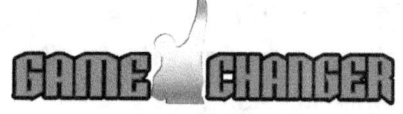

Chapter 7 – Your Fat Loss Questions Answered

Q: How Many Meals Should I Eat Per Day?

A: You may have heard the advice to eat 6 small meals a day, every 2-3 hours, to "speed up the metabolism." The truth is, meal frequency has very little (if any) effect on fat loss. It's the total sum of food you eat each day that's most important. Space out your food into the number of meals that best suit your lifestyle

Q: Does It Matter WHEN I Eat?

A: This concept is similar to the question above. *When* you eat your food has very little effect on your health, weight, and body composition. The most important thing is the total quality and quantity of your food, not the timing.

Eating breakfast in the morning might keep you fuller during the day, but you don't *have* to have it. You can even eat food right before going to bed. Your body doesn't stop digesting food or burning calories just because you are resting. As long as you do not eat too many calories, you won't suffer any ill effects from eating foods at specific times.

Q: How Quickly Should I Lose Weight?

A: Anyone can lose 10lbs in two weeks with a starvation diet, but that is not a healthy solution. Losing weight slowly produces the best long-term results. We advise losing about 0.5-1% of your body weight per week, so for a 150lb person this amounts to 0.75lbs-1.5lbs per week.

Your nutrition needs to fit a lifestyle. If you try to lose fat with an approach that you cannot see yourself doing a year from now, then it is probably the wrong approach. Crash dieting can cause lean muscle loss, fatigue, and psychological distress. If you are resistance training, you may even put on lean muscle, so it's possible your weight won't decrease much at all, but you will look and feel better.

Q: Why does my body weight change so much from day-to-day?

A: The scale number fluctuates based on what you ate recently, changes in hormones, hydration, recent sodium intake, and other factors. Your menstrual cycle can increase your weight for a whole week each month. You can eat a large meal, or go to the bathroom, and it can change your scale weight by several pounds. The good news is these fluctuations are temporary, and aren't preventing your fat loss.

It's important to view the changes in your body weight from week-to-week and month-to-month, rather than day-to-day. Weigh yourself multiple times a week if you're trying to lose body fat, and look at your weekly average.

Q: What foods should I NEVER have? What food should I ALWAYS have?

A: No individual food makes you gain weight, and no specific food can burn body fat. The TOTAL calories and nutrients you eat throughout the whole day are responsible for how you look. There is no such thing as a healthy or unhealthy food, there are only healthy or unhealthy diets or habits.

Q: How do I fix specific "trouble" areas of my body?

A: You can't target specific body parts to lose fat. You need to lose body fat all over, and eventually you'll lose it from specific areas. There will be spots on your body where the fat is last to leave, even as you lose weight.

There is no natural way to prioritize where you lose fat, no matter what food you eat or exercise you do. For example, if you want to lose body fat only from your stomach, you can't do that by training your abs every day. You need to lose body fat with proper diet and exercise, and eventually you'll lose fat from your stomach, even if that's the last place you lose it.

With strength training you can build up muscles to improve how they look. Building lean muscle mass gives you tone and definition. But if this muscle is covered in body fat, the definition is harder to see.

Q: If I eat "clean" during the week, can I eat whatever I want on the weekends?

One of the biggest reasons for failed fat loss is inconsistency. People often tell us "I hardly eat, yet I can't lose any weight." When we examine a full week of their nutrition, this doesn't turn out to be the case. Usually, their diets are good during the work week, but their weekend habits are very different, and this negates the hard work from the week.

Let's look at a tangible example. A woman maintains her body weight on 2,200 calories a day (this is just an example, not a generalization), so she eats 1,700 calories each day during the week to try and lose fat.

On the weekends, she rewards herself with a few alcoholic drinks one night, and goes out to eat and orders a large meal on another night. If she eats 3,500 calories each night of the weekend (something that isn't difficult when eating out and drinking enough alcohol) her average calorie intake for the week is still at 2,200. No wonder she can't lose body fat.

Good nutrition needs to be a full-time commitment. It doesn't need to be brutal and restrictive, but it must be consistent.

Q: How can I lose weight during the holidays? What if I'm always busy?

A: No matter what time of year it is, there will ALWAYS be parties, events, and holidays presenting challenges. The summer is filled with barbecues and vacations, the winter has Christmas and New Years. Year-round there are birthday parties, family dinners, ballgames, weddings, anniversaries, work outings, graduations, religious celebrations, nights out with friends, eating out at favorite restaurants, and countless other events.

There will never be a perfect time to get in shape, and you'll always be busy. If you want to overcome these challenges, you need to make your health and fitness a priority in your life.

Q: I exercise and I eat right, how come I can't lose weight?

A: You are probably not eating as little food as you think, and there's something you can do to figure this out. Log all the food you eat for an entire week. One of two things will happen:

1. You'll notice you eat more food than you thought
2. You'll finally lose weight because you made better choices over the week

Several studies show that many overweight individuals actually under-report how much food they intake. When people track their meals, their true diet comes to light. One study suggests the more overweight people are, the greater the chance they will misreport their diets. Another study shows some subjects under-reporting their food by over 2,000 calories a day! Some people consciously lie about their diets, but it is also very common for people to *forget* about food they eat. We cannot pinpoint the exact reasons that people misrepresent their diets, but we do know it's one of the obstacles you'll face, no matter how truthful and accurate you think you are. Fitness is not just about the body. Emotions and intellect play just as much a part in the process.

Q: I binged over the past few days. Is my diet ruined?

A: Absolutely not. How much could a poor week of eating slow down your progress? Maybe a week, or two, or maybe three weeks at the most? Don't you plan to keep your progress and good health beyond the date in which you would've originally reached your goals?

Maybe now you hit your goal body weight on June 1st instead of May 1st. Maybe now you fit into your old clothes in the winter rather than in the fall. Maybe now you can stop taking health medications after 10 years instead of 9 1/2.

A small step backwards is no reason to give up on your goals, especially when your health (and possibly your life) is on the line. You are human, you will slip up, and that's perfectly normal. Unless you lock yourself in a safe house with limited food, you WILL deviate from your plan from time to time.

Keeping with good nutritional habits is not like playing a game or competition. Just because you have a misstep doesn't mean you've lost. Having good nutrition 80% of the time is better than having it 0% of the time.

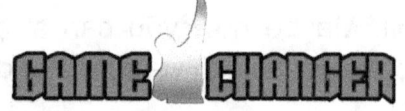

Chapter 8: How To Choose The Right Program To Help You Get Back Into Your Skinny Jeans

If you are thinking about hiring a personal trainer or coach, here are our four recommendations:

Recommendation # 1: Make a commitment to yourself and invest in a quality program with a proven track record of results. Do this as soon as possible. The longer you wait, the further away you will be from achieving your goals.

Recommendation # 2: List your objectives. Do you want to workout at a big box gym, where trainers are just working for a paycheck and get mediocre-to-average results? Or do you want to get the best results possible by going to a results focused facility that guarantees results, like ours?

Recommendation # 3: Ask questions. The best way to determine if a program is successful is to ask specific questions, and listen carefully to the answers. Here are a few questions we suggest you ask:

1) Do you have written success stories from moms who've joined your program?

2) How many days a week do you recommend I train?

3) What is your training philosophy when it comes to training busy moms like me?

4) What training and experience do you have in training and coaching other moms?

5) What type of training do you do during each session?

Recommendation # 4: Once you have found a program you think will give you the best results, ask to sign up for a free consultation. During this consultation, the trainer or coach should listen to your needs and wants. They should learn your goals, what things have worked for you in the past, what hasn't worked, and let you know exactly what you should expect when you join.

By following the information in this book, you'll make an informed decision when choosing a program that's right for you. If you want to join a cheap, unproven program, there are probably plenty of low-cost options available in your area. But if you want to join a top-notch program with a proven track record to help busy moms just like you - then I invite you to call us.

I'll be happy to answer your questions - tell you how our membership works - or schedule you for a free consultation - without any obligation. To reach us, call our facility 973-376-9003 and ask for Joe Meglio or, if you prefer, e-mail us at Joe@gamechangergym.com, and we will be happy to answer your questions.

Here's one last point: we know many moms are skeptical about getting involved in a fitness program. That's why at GameChanger, we guarantee our work. That's right, we fully guarantee your results. If you aren't completely satisfied with your results, we'll refund you every single penny.

As a matter of fact, add this additional question to the list above: (6) "Do you guarantee your work?" Not all fitness programs do and it's important that you have this information before you make your decision.

Thank you very much for reading *The Skinny Jeans Solution For Busy Moms*.

About the Authors

Joe Meglio is the owner of GameChanger Strength & Performance in Springfield, New Jersey. He is a published author of the Amazon best selling book *No Gym, No Time, No Problem* and also the author of *The Parent's Guide to Strength Training for Baseball.*

Joe was named the first ever STACK.com Expert of the Month and in 2011 he was voted the # 1 Rising Star in the Fitness Industry by Fitnessbusiness-interviews.com. He has been featured in Today's Man Magazine, STACK Magazine, EliteFTS.com, ESPN Page 2 & the Staten Island Advance.

Rob Riccobono is a strength & nutrition coach at GameChanger Strength & Performance. He has directly worked with hundres of busy moms on their nutrition, helping them lose weight and transform their bodies.

Rob is an ACSM-certified personal trainer & a Certified Nutrition Coach from Precision Nutrition, the largest private nutrition coaching and research company in the world.

Reference Page

Chapter 2
"You can't build a perkier, rounder, or sexier _anything_ without building muscle."- Nick Tumminello, "Strength Training for Fat Loss"

Chapter 3
Sugar sweetened beverages and long-term weight gain- Malik VS, et al. Curr Diab Rep. 2012. "Sweeteners and Risk of Obesity and Type 2 Diabetes: The Role of Sugar-Sweetened Beverages."
http://www.ncbi.nlm.nih.gov/m/pubmed/22289979/

Alcohol stimulates hunger- Hetherington MM, et al. Physiol Behav. 2001. "Stimulation of appetite by alcohol."
http://www.ncbi.nlm.nih.gov/pubmed/11714490

Moderate alcohol consumption increased subsequent food intake- Schrieks IC, et al. Appetite. 2015. "Moderate alcohol consumption stimulates food intake and food reward of savoury foods."
http://www.ncbi.nlm.nih.gov/pubmed/25636235

Weight loss from water- Dennis EA, et al.

Obesity (Silver Spring). 2010. "Water consumption increases weight loss during a hypocaloric diet intervention in middle-aged and older adults." http://www.ncbi.nlm.nih.gov/m/pubmed/19661958/

Water, women and their mood- Dennis EA, et al. Obesity (Silver Spring). 2010. "Water consumption increases weight loss during a hypocaloric diet intervention in middle-aged and older adults." http://www.ncbi.nlm.nih.gov/pubmed/25963107

Coffee and decreased risk of Type II Diabetes- Akash MS1, Rehman K2, Chen S3. "Effects of coffee on type 2 diabetes mellitus." http://www.ncbi.nlm.nih.gov/pubmed/24984989

Caffeine slightly boosts metabolism- Belza A1, Toubro S, Astrup A. "The effect of caffeine, green tea and tyrosine on thermogenesis and energy intake." http://www.ncbi.nlm.nih.gov/pubmed/17882140

Aspartame safety- Butchko HH, et al. Regul Toxicol Pharmacol. 2001. "Aspartame: scientific evaluation in the postmarketing period." http://www.ncbi.nlm.nih.gov/m/pubmed/1175452

Chapter 4
High protein diets, more weight loss- Wycherley TP, et al. Am J Clin Nutr. 2012. "Effects of energy-restricted high-protein, low-fat compared with standard-protein, low-fat diets: a meta-analysis of randomized controlled trials." http://www.ncbi.nlm.nih.gov/pubmed/23097268

High protein diets, blood pressure and blood sugar- Dong JY, et al. Br J Nutr. 2013. "Effects of high-protein diets on body weight, glycaemic control, blood lipids and blood pressure in type 2 diabetes: meta-analysis of randomised controlled trials." http://www.ncbi.nlm.nih.gov/pubmed/23829939

Chapter 5
Fruits and vegetables prevent illness- Rui Hai Liu, Sep 2003. "Health benefits of fruit and vegetables are from additive and synergistic combinations of phytochemicals."http://ajcn.nutrition.org/content/78/3/517S.full

Fructose concerns from fruit- Alan Aragon, January 2010. "The Bitter Truth of Fructose Alarmism."

http://www.alanaragonblog.com/2010/01/29/the-bitter-truth-about-fructose-alarmism

Lower risk of obesity in women, fruit consumption- Rautiainen S, et al. J Nutr. 2015. "Higher Intake of Fruit, but Not Vegetables or Fiber, at Baseline Is Associated with Lower Risk of Becoming Overweight or Obese in Middle-Aged and Older Women of Normal BMI at Baseline."
http://www.ncbi.nlm.nih.gov/pubmed/25934663

Chapter 8
Misreporting your diet- Heitmann BL[1], Lissner L. "Dietary underreporting by obese individuals-- is it specific or non-specific?".
http://www.ncbi.nlm.nih.gov/pubmed/7580640

Underreporting food by thousands of calories- Buhl KM[1], Gallagher D, Hoy K, Matthews DE, Heymsfield SB. "Unexplained disturbance in body weight regulation: diagnostic outcome assessed by doubly labeled water and body composition analyses in obese patients reporting low energy intakes."
http://www.ncbi.nlm.nih.gov/pubmed/7594141